Suggestions from the Other Side

Pearls of Wisdom and Resources for PA and NP Students and New Grads

By:
Kelsey Riebel, PA-C

Visit www.midlevelsos.com to access the template and list downloads.

ISBN : 978-1-7342341-0-7

Table of Contents

Preface

Forget all the facts and memorization – well, don't forget it you're going to need it. Just set it aside for now. This is not a book about how to diagnose, treat, or counsel your soon to be patients. You've already done the work to learn all that stuff and now you need some practical and actionable templates, lists, resources, and general tips and tricks to help you get through your first year of practice. You've undoubtedly had a lot of experience on clinical rotations and you may feel completely ready to take on the world, but things are different on the outside. Consider what I suggest, but feel free to take what you read and make it entirely your own. That's the purpose of this book: to help you feel more prepared and organized before hitting the clinic for real. I hope it will serve as a launch pad from which you can create your own finely tuned system that works best for you. I've been in your shoes and have learned a lot along the way. Let me guide you and help you to be your best self.

When I was preparing to begin my first job after PA school, I made lists of the most common diagnoses along with the most current treatment guidelines, reviewed all my BLS and ACLS algorithms, and was generally having trouble sleeping at night due to all the anxiety and excitement. I wanted to be the most prepared that I could possibly be, so that I would provide great patient care (and not look like an idiot).

If you've recently graduated or are going back to primary care after working in a specialty, I'm betting you're doing all the same things I described above, because let's face it: we're all a little type A in this profession. I looked for resources to help me feel more prepared, but I just couldn't find any. Most of the resources out there consist of specific diagnosis or treatment guidelines, but not information about how to survive the day-to-day work. This book is a compilation of all the resources I have discovered and practices I have developed while being in the trenches the last three years. I currently use these to help me be more efficient and feel less like a basket case everyday. This book won't give you all the medical information you'll need to know, but it will give you a ton of great resources where you can find the best and most concise information to help you in your busy practice. It will also give you several templates to make your life easier and your work go faster.

I haven't been out of PA school long, but I think that puts me in the best position to write this book for you. I have been in practice long enough to develop some useful strategies, templates, and routines that I wish I had known when I graduated, but it hasn't been so long that I've forgotten how it feels to be standing square in your shoes. Hopefully, the resources and experience I can provide will act as the lifeboat to rescue you from the riptide and undercurrent that can sometimes make up the world of medicine. That's the goal. Feel free to take these ideas and change them to suit your needs. This book was created to be delivered in a PDF format, so that you can print directly from this download, copy and paste text into EHR templates, etc. for quick and easy application.

The "Master Sheet" template will be referenced several times throughout this book. It is a template that I created to help me be more efficient and thorough during a visit. It also helps the patient understand (and remember) what changes were made or what the next steps will be. It is structured similar to an office visit note. There are sections including: the chief complaint, HPI, preventive care, immunizations, pertinent physical exam findings, and the assessment and plan. I use this portion of the template to jot down my own notes and then use them to write the note later. This is especially helpful if I get busy and the note doesn't get done until the end of the day. There is also a section to the right that is meant to be torn off and given to the patient as a summary. Some EHRs offer a visit summary to print out and give, but I never had this luxury and the EHR summaries I have received as a patient haven't been all that helpful. The patient section includes: the diagnosis, treatment plan, medication changes, other instructions, and when to follow up. See the template near the end of the book for more details.

Before we get started let me first say this. I will use the term midlevel to encompass both NP and PA professionals throughout this book. If this offends you I apologize in advance, but if so go ahead and honestly get over it. I only use the term because it is easier to talk about both professions at the same time this way. I in no way intend to start a debate about titles. If you are a midlevel, titles clearly weren't the point for your degree, so let's not get hung up on it. Thanks in advance.

5 Common Problems in Practice

In this section, I'll discuss the most common problems I have encountered in primary care. Below each problem is my proposed solution to try in your own practice. If these solutions are implemented from the beginning, it may save you some frustrations in the future.

1. Patients try to address too many problems for the time slot allowed.

This is a common problem that all providers face, especially with corporations shortening appointment times and pushing productivity measures such as relative value units (RVUs), etc. To help make your visit more focused, and therefore more efficient, ask nursing staff to have the patient list his or her top two most concerning problems that they wish to address today. After these are written down on your Master Sheet template in the appropriate section, the nurse should ask about any other problems concerning the patient. These should be placed in a separate section and the patient should be given the opportunity to schedule for these prior to you entering the room. This way the patient feels the other issues will be taken care of in the near future, but they also understand that is not going to be today.

2. Patients don't know what meds they take and they have different medication lists at your primary care office, the urgent care, at the specialist's office, and the hospital. This makes management hard and keeps you chasing your tail.

During my time in the hospital and the primary care clinic, it became clear very quickly that most patients do not know what meds they are taking or what they are for. At each visit with you an up to date medication list should be printed and given to the patient with any changes to the list included and highlighted. It would be even better if this could be scaled down to fit in his or her wallet or purse, or if the patient prefers she can take a picture of it to keep on her phone in case she loses the paper copy. Any changes should also be written clearly on their take home slip (see the Master Sheet template). It is nearly impossible to manage chronic disease well if we don't know what the patient is taking and if the patient doesn't understand what he should be taking. How can we know what changes to make? Bringing a bag of meds can sometimes be helpful (and patients often do this), but it is very time consuming in the clinic and burdensome to the patient. It also increases the risk that they may lose some of their medicine in the process.

3. Patients can't summarize office visits and generally don't understand what happened or what to do next.

Patients often seem to follow what is going on during conversation in the exam room, but then when asked to repeat the plan, change in treatment, or action they agreed to take 3 seconds ago, there are often only crickets heard in the room. This isn't any fault of the patient. Generally, a lot gets discussed during the visit and we usually forget (or don't feel we have time to) slow down when we explain or sometimes accidentally use words we forget that the general public doesn't understand. A quick summary written down for the patient can take less than a minute and can significantly increase compliance and patient satisfaction. It also helps consolidate the visit in your own mind so that you can be more efficient when writing your note. Additionally, it can help prevent you from forgetting to order something you discussed during the visit. Sometimes, the patient can even help you remember to order something you forgot and this will save you time later on the phone or in the chart to correct it. Everyone wins.

4. Visits can be too focused and the patient may not make it back for a general examination of their record. It is important to think about the patient as a whole and not only the problem they bring on a particular day. This can be more difficult than it sounds, especially on busy days. Are they on the right medications for their comorbidities? Are they up to date on immunizations and screenings? Do they need lab?

When I'm pressed for time (because who isn't?) the visit is often hyper-focused on the specific problem they came in for. This isn't bad all of the time, but if the patient doesn't come in for at least an annual review of their comorbidities and med review these important tasks can fall through the cracks. I created the Master Sheet template to help with this by creating a quick snapshot of the patient. Theoretically, the electronic health record should be used for this snapshot, but I often find that things aren't in the place they ought to be, comorbidities are missing from their problem list, etc. It just never worked well for me. Nursing staff can use the Master Sheet template to jot down their pertinent past medical history, immunizations (simply whether they are up to date or not), and screenings they may be due for, so they can be seen at a glance when we're in the room with the patient. This allows us to discuss these issues with the patient quickly while we're there so they won't get behind on these standards of care. Alternatively, you can begin implementing pieces of the Master Sheet template into your note, and then can copy and paste these snapshots at the beginning or end of each new note (with appropriate updates) if this makes things run more smoothly and quickly for you.

5. Providers look up the same information several times. This helps with memorization, but it is very inefficient in a very time limited environment.

I have 500+ continuing medical education (CME) hours accumulated on UpToDate® as I am writing this. I look up information constantly. Usually, I do this on UpToDate®, because it is super easy to search just like Google. Also, there are concise summaries below the very detailed information above. With all the information we are expected to know and have memorized, I am extra paranoid that I will forget an important detail, or remember something incorrectly and make a mistake that could harm a patient. Resources, people. We have to use them, because there is just too much information. Aside from the quantity of information, it is constantly changing. I always heard this in PA school, but it has changed faster than I ever thought it would. I used to feel inadequate looking up information all of the time, because I felt like I had to be the omniscient being that patients sometimes think we are. Now, I attribute my continual research to the fact that I strive to be a conscientious provider who does the best I can for my patients. I'd rather be researching too much than too little. It is so dang time consuming, though. I waste a lot of time looking up the same things I looked up last week; ESPECIALLY in primary care, because the breadth of problems and disease processes that we are responsible for is so stinking wide. If I did the exact same thing every day and counseled on the exact same topic during every patient encounter then I wouldn't need to look up information as much. However, because I see diabetes, heart disease, women's health, men's health, musculoskeletal problems, lung disease, acute lacerations, neurological disease, mental health issues, skin disorders, liver disease, and drug addiction among others, sometimes I forget the minutiae of what I looked up last week. Will you forgive me? For this reason, I think it helps with efficiency to have algorithms and tables on speed dial. They are quick, clear, and easy to act on. We will discuss specific resources where you can find the best tables and algorithms later on.

Other Suggestions

Before we move on to the most useful resources, templates, and lists to help you in your first year or two, I wanted to briefly touch on a few nuggets of wisdom I feel will be helpful for you to read. Below is a small collection of wisdom that I've acquired on the job and in the trenches. These points have been helpful for me to remember in order to be able to continue to show up day after day.

1. "Cut yourself some slack in the first year." This advice was passed on to me by a friend who had heard it from a preceptor. I think it is easy to agree with, but hard to actually do. There is a huge learning curve after graduation and we don't have a residency, so it's understandable to struggle a little at first just as most first year residents do. They have way more support built into residency, so I think we're doing bomb surviving without it. More than surviving, I believe that we're flourishing.

2. Ask your colleagues questions. I always felt inadequate when doing this at first, but now I understand that was just silly. Patients will appreciate that you're using all the resources possible to help make the best decision for them and your physician and midlevel colleagues alike will respect you for recognizing and admitting your own limitations. Don't worry. You will need to ask far fewer questions every day of practice.

3. I don't wear a white coat. I have colleagues who do wear a white coat, and some studies actually demonstrate that patients may prefer it, but I tend to disagree (whether I have a study to back me up or not). I like being casual (with my dress and demeanor) in the room, because I think it makes patients more comfortable overall and more willing to discuss uncomfortable or embarrassing issues with you. That's not to

say you shouldn't dress professionally, but I just leave off the white coat. For God's sake there is a diagnosis to support the fact that the white coat makes people nervous! (That is white coat hypertension for those of you who didn't study.) I sometimes even try to posture myself casually. If the patient is in the chair next to the exam table, I might roll my chair next to the exam table, put my feet on the step of the exam table (not with my feet crossed and lounging, but feet flat, and knees bent) and I'll write on my paper on the exam table. This is also helpful if he is hard of hearing ("HOH"), because you're positioned closer to him.

4. I don't chart in the room. I've received a lot of pressure to do so, and many have said, "You might as well get used to it, because you're going to have to eventually to get all your work done." A lot of people think multitasking makes you faster and more efficient, but I would argue the opposite. For example, I am much less efficient when I am thinking in medical jargon while typing my note, but then make my brain switch gears to speak more plainly and personably to the patient sitting in front of me. If you're trying to complete a note as the patient interview is taking place, you're going to be switching gears at least ten times and probably more. Also, I strongly believe based on patient comments that they prefer us to jot notes down on our paper rather than type in the computer. It's much more personable and I can spend more time looking the patient in the eye when they're telling me about something personal. They can feel this difference. Also, if you're doing the note in the room you are typing, which is rookie mistake #1. Typing is much slower than dictation.

Doing the note just after the patient leaves allows me to use a dictation software like Dragon® back at my desk. My employer pays for this service. It seriously cuts down the time it takes me to write a note, and I consider myself a speedy typer. I have found that colleagues who don't use the dictation software are frequently behind on notes. Computers in the exam room are helpful for discussing information with the patient like recent labs or medication changes. Instead of taking time to log into the computer in the room, I tend to jot labs down in two columns: one column under the heading of "WNL" and another column with the heading "ABN" for abnormal. Under the "ABN" column, I write down the specifics to discuss with the patient. When I'm in the room I expand on the normal labs (ie. CBC and CMP) by saying: "electrolytes, kidneys, liver, and blood counts were all normal." If there are more extensive labs to discuss I just print out the report to save time. Sorry rainforest. I also always have nursing print a current medication list. I particularly like this printed out, because then I can write notes next to each drug, for example, if they're taking a different dose, if we plan to change the dose or frequency, or if we're going to discontinue it altogether. I can write quick notes next to each one reminding me to change it in the computer after our visit. Sometimes nursing staff can help make these changes to their chart as well, so this can also save you time.

5. When trying to prioritize what to do first after I leave the room, I have a checklist that looks like this:

1. Labs and Xray
2. Meds
3. Problem
4. Bill
5. Note
6. Referrals

I use the checklist to ensure I don't forget anything. My clinic has lab and X-ray in the same building, so I order these first because they are what the patient does immediately after they leave the exam room. Then, I immediately order any meds or make any changes to their current medications, because we also have pharmacy on-site and I don't want them to be waiting on me to put in the order when I'm in another patient room (for God knows how long). The problem category is just a reminder to select the item that we addressed from their current problem list or add a new problem for billing purposes. This helps to speed up ordering labs and meds, so that the indication populates in the drop down window and can be selected from a list instead of searching for it every time. The billing portion is just a single click and is done anytime, but I usually do it just after entering or selecting the problem so that I don't forget it altogether. Next to last is the note. It helps me to do this before any referrals are placed, because I have just gathered and summarized all my thoughts into the note. Often, the reason for referral can be copied and pasted from the note. Your EHR and or clinic will probably be a little different, but not entirely. Doing the note and referrals last allows me to put these on hold if I get behind or if other patients are already in a room waiting for me. At the end of the morning or afternoon session I may have a few notes to catch up on, but generally there are not many. I would much rather do my notes in peace without interruptions or extra stress knowing that a patient (or several) are waiting on me to finish my note before seeing them.

6. Make people stay out of your office and have your own private office if at all possible. I have countless distractions and interruptions every day, because I share my office with the nurse I work with. Usually the person interrupting us doesn't need anything important, and she doesn't need to speak in person, but she just comes to chat. One small question turns into a long conversation about her husband or kid and I'm left trying to figure out where I was going with my last sentence. It might seem nice to build up some camaraderie with coworkers, but this can be done at specific break times. My work takes me all day, so if I'm slowed down by nonsense interruptions mama ain't happy, because it means I'm getting home late. One day I told the nurse who shares my office I was in a negativity funk and was trying to turn my

mood around and be positive. No joke, almost immediately at least five people marched in one right after the other to complain about something, usually work, a supervisor, or a coworker. This created 2-3 hours of negativity and time we all won't get back. Some people just live to create drama and I hate being forced to be around it. Let's put out positive vibes people. You get more positivity back that way.

7. Write notes that are really useful. This sounds intuitive, but surprisingly most people do not do this. Most either use only pre-populated data from the chart, or they type one to two lines in the HPI and one or two words in the assessment and plan. I don't know how your memory is, but mine is about as good as an ant's. I actually don't know if ants have great memories or not, but it seems like it would be subpar given their tiny brains. Do ants have brains? The point is that if you can dictate a thorough HPI and assessment and plan you'll be much better off when the patient comes in for the chief complaint of "test results." "Crap, what did we order? Why the hell did I order that?" If you can write down your thought process and even possible next steps (especially if you've looked something up), it will save you loads of time when they come for follow up and you won't sound like you have no idea what's going on, because that sucks. Also, your coworkers won't hate you if they see your patient on follow up.

8. Sometimes it is okay to leave a little work to do the next day. When I first started, I would get all my work done before going home, and this is a good habit to get into in the beginning. Later, as my comfort level increased and I could estimate my time to complete tasks, I started leaving a little work for in the morning prior to the start of clinic. I'm usually pooped at the end of the day, so my concentration on notifications (labs, reports, etc.) is diminished. When I'm rejuvenat-

ed in the morning, I can make better decisions faster regarding these notifications. Also, the more time I have in the evening with my family the better. Additionally, I am neurotically early every day (about 30-40 minutes before clinic starts). Leaving just a smidge of work to do in the morning helps me get my juices flowing and prevents me from sitting there twiddling my thumbs. I usually try not to leave more than half a page worth of notifications and only one or two notes. Notifications are less irritating in the morning than notes are, so I try to get all the notes done on the "date of service." It can be difficult to remember all the details of an encounter you had yesterday.

9. Chief complaints can be helpful, but a lot of the time they are useless and completely wrong. This all depends on the patient and the scheduler. Sometimes the patient is too embarrassed to say the real reason they want to come in, or sometimes the person scheduling just doesn't pay attention or ask the right questions. The point is this: I used to get all worried about preparing for as many patients as possible prior to the session, so I felt like I had a good plan and had plenty of time to look up and print patient information to give out. What I found was that I was spending a ton of extra time doing this preparation and then the patient would either no-show, reschedule, or be there for something completely different. It all ends up being wasted time, because even if I saved the info I prepared beforehand I would still have to review it again just before his rescheduled visit. I would also get labs and imaging results confused, because I had looked up so many at once. Now, I just wait for the patient to show up before scanning the chart and then quickly looking up what I need just before going into the room. This takes just a couple of minutes usually, and the info is super fresh in your mind to regurgitate to the patient. No time is wasted on things they're actually not there for or on problems that weren't serious enough to show up for.

10. Form a great network of colleagues. This doesn't mean schmoozing at events or CME conferences. What I mean is this: be a positive presence in all your affairs at work. Be on time, a self-starter, get work done in a timely manner, etc. It's true that every day is an interview. Most job offers will come without seeking and applying for positions. If you've built a great network, someone will call you and offer it to you without you knowing about the open position, applying for it, or even interviewing for it. You may even get offers from people you don't know solely based on what someone has heard about you. This is not an exaggeration. It has happened to me. People talk. Give them something good to say and you'll reap benefits later. Working in the hospital was very helpful to me when building my network. You end up working with A LOT of different physicians, midlevels, and nurses who all can be potential bridges to new opportunities.

11. Don't forget about prescriber information summaries for help on how to start, stop, or switch medications. This is especially helpful for birth control (Nexplanon®, IUDs, Nuvaring®). See the appropriate brand's website to find this. Usually, websites with information for providers (including the prescribing information) has the letters "hcp" somewhere in the web address. I normally just search the brand plus "prescribing information" in a search engine.

12. Join an email list to get current medical news and up to date guidelines. Some of the emails I am signed up to receive include Physician's First Watch, ACP Hospitalist Weekly, and Medscape Family Medicine. I didn't know about these until a year or so into practice. They are very good at keeping you up to date with the newest research and articles. I have found that they all generally have much of the same information, so to reduce your email burden I recommend choosing one and no more than that.

13. Exercise and get away from work during the day. Having patients scheduled all day can be daunting. At times I feel I am chained to my computer from dawn to dusk. At first, I was so concerned with getting my notes done that I would hardly take a break to snarf my lunch down. Now, I get as much done as I am able before a certain time and when at all possible (which is most days), I go for a walk outside. The sun, wind, and exercise do wonders to help reset my mind and attitude for the afternoon session. Without it I would lose my sanity. Coworkers have attested to this.

"The Curbsiders" internal medicine podcast does a great job highlighting that mental health is an important topic to discuss and they make a concerted effort to promote this throughout their show. The first part of each episode (about 10 minutes or so) is usually a fun discussion about de-stressing and wellness strategies, including recent book recommendations, best movies or TV shows, and other ways to balance your life and be your best self. Often, they have residents and others on the show to discuss their own frustrations with medicine and the institutions they work for and ways to deal with these pains. They often ask the expert what his or her most valuable failure is and lift this up as a learning opportunity instead of something to be ashamed of. I think often in medicine we feel we must be perfectionists (I know this is something that I struggle with every day - we're dealing with people's lives for God's sake). Perfection is not something that is attainable, so when mistakes are made it is best to share them, so that everyone can learn from and be improved by it, instead of hiding from and feeling ashamed of it.

Book Resources

Next, let's discuss specific resources you can begin exploring to see how they can improve your practice, make you more efficient, and feel more prepared for the clinic. The resources we'll discuss are ones that I personally use. These books sit on my desk, the websites are saved to my desktop, and the apps are currently on my phone. I have acquired these resources from years of experience and via recommendations from colleagues and teachers in school and on the job. The lists of materials for common procedures near the end of the book were derived entirely from the sticky notes on my desk that I use regularly to help me remember what I need. Let's begin.

The Sanford Guide to Antimicrobial Therapy 2019 by David Gilbert, M.D., et al.

I have learned to use this resource a lot. I first used it when I was working in the hospital, but I also use it a lot in primary care. The section I use most often is the "Antibacterial Activity Spectra." This section provides easy to read tables for a quick reference to check antibiotic coverage for a specific organism. The tables list specific drugs and are organized by class. It helps you to quickly identify which antibiotic will be most effective and which are first-line, second-line, etc. For example, I use it when I get a weird bug back on a urine culture to ensure the antibiotic I had previously selected empirically is adequate coverage for the organism. All of the pharmacists I know use this resource a lot.

Another useful tool in this book is the table of specific diagnoses (organized by location of infection) with recommended first-line treatment along with alternatives. Dosing recommendations are also included. There is another great table with recommended duration of therapy, and it is organized by site and diagnosis. This is essential to reference often to avoid prescribing too many days worth of therapy (or not enough) for the specific indication. This helps us to be better antibiotic stewards and to ensure that the infection is adequately treated.

To add to the long list of tables (which are concise and easy to read and digest quickly), there is another table titled "Pharmacologic Features." This table is great for identifying features of certain drugs such as, route of administration and time to peak serum concentration among many other details. The half-life information is found in another table titled "Dosage of Antimicrobial Drugs in Adult Patients with Renal Impairment" (although I usually look this up on UpToDate®, because it is so easy and quick to find there). There is also a half-life time for normal renal function in this same table. Often, patients will ask if a particular drug is still in their system when discussing side effects, for example. The other time I've found it most helpful to know the half-life of a drug is when a negative UDS is discovered when the patient was supposed to have been taking a particular medication (ie. controlled substance). A negative UDS combined with a patient who says he or she is still taking it may indicate diversion. When the half-life is multiplied by 5 you have the approximate time that most would consider it to be "out of your system." I use this number to determine if the UDS should be positive or negative. When in doubt, especially if you're considering discontinuing the controlled substance and therefore accusing your patient of suspicious and prohibited behavior, it is always necessary to send the sample for a confirmatory test.

Another table describes appropriate pediatric dosing and this makes it easy to do the quick math for pediatric dosing based on the child's weight. There is also a really great drug-drug interaction table when needed. And if you thought that was all you would ever need, you'll find another table with generic drugs matched with their trade names, which can be helpful especially if you don't have Internet access for some reason. Otherwise, I just quickly type it into UpToDate® and usually the generic drug populates. If you're looking for the trade name from a generic drug on UpToDate®, you can search the generic and then click on the section for brand name and it is quickly displayed. All in all, The Sanford Guide is a trusted pharmacy and clinic resource, and because all the pharmacists I know trust it, I trust it.

Injection Techniques in Musculoskeletal Medicine A Practical Manual for Clinicians in Primary and Secondary Care by Stephanie Saunders and Steve Longworth.

This is a new resource I was introduced to by a co-worker. This particular co-worker is a nurse practitioner that previously worked in the ER setting and loves procedures, so I definitely trusted her recommendation on this one. The book starts by discussing the evidence behind injections, as well as current controversies, and the rationale of several therapies including corticosteroids and local anesthetics. Additionally, it discusses the most common potential side effects to consider as well as the costs related to each therapy. This is great for casual reading if you have any administrative time not consumed by paperwork and charting, but for everyday practical use there is a section for "Upper Limb Injections" and another for "Lower Limb Injections." There is also a spinal injection section, but I don't use this in primary care.

The upper and lower limb sections are great, because they offer very practical and concise information, including the specific target for the injection, the equipment you'll need (size of syringe, needle size, as well as amounts and concentration of the steroid and anesthetic), appropriate technique, aftercare instructions, and clinical pearls (such as how to differentiate certain diagnoses on exam). And if you think it can't get better people, there are pictures. There are hand-sketched pictures with bones, muscles, tendons, and bursae, but there are also pictures of the injection location on real humans with flesh. They have drawn in the anatomic markers that you'll be looking and feeling for and superimposed these on top of the photo of a real human. This is very helpful when trying to find markers on a real patient. At the beginning of each chapter you'll also find the most beneficial examination techniques for the major joints.

Lastly, the purchase of this text also includes a virtual component which includes over fifty video clips, other animations, and self-testing resources to help perfect your skills.

Clinician's Guide to Laboratory Medicine by Samir P. Desai, M.D.

This resource was suggested to me by a preceptor of mine on my internal medicine rotation. I felt, and still feel, that he is one of the most thoughtful, intelligent, compassionate, and thorough PAs I have ever worked with. I was grateful to receive this book title as a recommendation from him, because I felt that if he used it and thought it was a great resource it definitely had to be. I have found it to be invaluable and super quick to reference.

The book is organized into a section of electrolyte and acid-base abnormalities at the beginning, then it is broken up into lab abnormalities sorted by systems (nephrology, hematology, gastroenterology, etc.). There are oodles of algorithms and I find this form of information to be one of the most clear and efficient ways to figure out your next step. In addition to these easy to use algorithms, they also offer more detailed information regarding their approach to each abnormality including potential etiologies for the abnormality and the next tests to help narrow your differential. There is a ton of valuable information in this book and I use it often in daily practice.

Instant Work-Ups by Theodore X. O'Connell

This is another great book recommended to me by a hospitalist NP co-worker. In addition to its great content within the book, there is also a code for online access. The book is organized into 78 of the most common problems primary care providers face. For each problem or diagnosis there is first a section with general information. There is a wealth of information in these sections, but it is also very concise. Next, each problem has a list of potential etiologies, important historical and physical exam features, suggested initial work-up, additional work-up, and then of course tables and algorithms as appropriate. There is also a list of references at the end of each section for further reading on the subject. Each section is usually only three pages or so. It is enough information to be a stand-alone resource, but is concise enough to consume quickly.

Pocket Primary Care 2nd Edition by Meghan M. Kiefer and Curtis R. Chong

In my experience, this book is a little bit more difficult to navigate than the others mentioned previously. Don't misunderstand me. It has a lot of helpful information, but the layout and abbreviations make it a little more difficult to read and determine your next steps quickly. I don't mean the usual abbreviations most clinicians use (well those are in there too), but I mean some serious shorthand in order to keep the sections and overall book small enough so that it can be carried in your pocket, hence the title. There are exactly 12.5 pages entirely dedicated to abbreviations. SIY WNT 2 BCM AN NTRPRTR 4 TH CIA DEF GT THS BK (Abbreviation in the back: So if you want to become an interpreter for the CIA definitely get this book.) Again, as I said it has great information it's just hard for me to digest quickly and maybe that's a fault of my own. Who knows? Each section has different information depending on the problem, and each problem is organized into larger sections defined by the system the problem is located in.

Normally, there are a few lines of information regarding each: general information, most common causes, pertinent history to obtain, important exam findings, initial work-up, recommended treatment, indications for referral, and follow-up if necessary. There are also tables and algorithms as appropriate. I did find their current screening guidelines and standardized classification systems and questionnaires to be very helpful [ie. NYHA/AHA Heart Failure Classification and International Prostate Symptom Score (IPSS), etc.].

Website Resources

All the websites in this section are currently on my desktop as active shortcuts, because I frequently use them. I find them to be invaluable and your computer desktop wouldn't be complete without them. I'll start with the ones I use the most. A list of all the websites can be found at the end of the book.

UpToDate®

This is hands down the most valuable all-in-one resource in my mind. I use it: Every. Single. Day. They offer a website and an app, and both are essentially identical information. Everywhere I've worked UpToDate® is paid for by the organization and therefore free for me to use. We also had access to this in PA school, although I didn't understand the immense power it contained until after graduation. If your employer doesn't already pay for a subscription, I'm sure it would be covered and considered reimbursable under your CME or other education allowance you have as part of your compensation package. The website is https://www.uptodate.com/home.

I describe it to others as a peer-reviewed and scholar trusted search engine like Google. All the docs I've worked with use it all the time and they do often make decisions with the information they find there. It is also a fantastic resource to find patient information handouts. I also recently discovered that there is a FREE patient site with printable handouts for the most common diagnoses that the patient can access on his or her own. The patient site is: www.patients.uptodate.com. There are two levels of patient information available to healthcare subscribers: "The Basics" and "Beyond the Basics." The former is a short overview of the topic and it aims to answer some of the most common patient questions related to it. The "Beyond the Basics" handout is a longer and more detailed summary with some medical terminology used. The free patient site provides all the "Beyond the Basics" information designed for patients. "The Basics" information is not included in this free content. This is a great quality and trusted resource for patients to get information regarding whatever diagnosis you've just given them. One approach to using this resource is to provide the patient with "The Basics" handout that only you have access to through your subscription, and then give them the website to go to and the topic to search in order to get more detailed information if they wish (which they can get on their own without the subscription).

As a provider, I use the subscriber content on a daily basis. I would almost bet I use it on an hourly basis. The articles are written by experts in the specific field and are peer-reviewed with references at the end of each entry. I use the app most frequently. When you type in a diagnosis that you want to explore, you first see a "Topic Outline." This provides quick access to specific sections that you may be looking for. When in a hurry, the "Summary & Recommendations" tab is the fastest way to get a concise overview of the pathophysiology, most common organism, clinical presentation, physical exam, imaging, labs, diagnosis, and treatment. If more detailed information is needed regarding the information in the summary section, you can quickly find those sections in the "Topic Outline" and get what you need. Additionally, you can search the text for a specific piece of information. For example, I have previously been curious about the incubation period of a certain organism, but don't have time to wade through all the super valuable information they have to offer on each subject. Instead, you can simply search "incubation period" in the specific article you've already found on Epstein Barr virus, for example, and it will quickly take you to the section where they discuss in the incubation period.

The most common topics I look up (mostly to double check myself given the chaos of any particular day in the clinic) are: suggested antibiotic and dosing for a specific indication, max dosing of a particular drug, pediatric dosing, drug side effects, drug half-life (under the "Pharmacodynamics and Pharmacokinetics" section), renal dosing, geriatric dosing, drug contraindications, pregnancy and breast-feeding implications, monitoring parameters, pricing, and brand names.

UpToDate® also offers a bookmark feature in order to quickly look up something you previously marked as important. Additionally, there are many calculators available such as CHA2DS2-VASc score, HAS-BLED bleeding risk score, cardiovascular risk assessment, unit conversions, creatinine-clearance calculator (Cockcroft-Gault), among many, many others.

The other feature I use most often is the "Drug Interactions" section, supported by Lexicomp®, a trusted pharmacist resource. You simply select your drugs to cross check and the system runs an analysis on the combination giving you a "Risk Rating" of A, B, C, D, or X. "A" correlates to "no interaction", "B" correlates to "no action needed", "C" correlates to "monitor therapy", "D" correlates to "modify regimen", and "X" correlates to "avoid combination".

Another great thing about UpToDate® is that you can sort your search results by: All, Adult, Pediatric, or Patient. Additionally, once you select your topic article, if you scroll to the very bottom of the outline you can find a section called "Graphics." I didn't know this for a long time. If there are any algorithms or tables that you know you have used before and you need to reference them quickly you can find them here.

The last thing I will say about UpToDate® is that not only is it a fantastic all-in-one resource for a busy clinical practice, it also is a great resource for CME credits. Every time you search something in Up-

ToDate®, it tracks the associated CME hours you can claim for it. It rewards you for expanding your knowledge on a topic when you see it in the clinic, which really helps with retention. It's no wonder they offer CME credits. To claim your credits (which I do almost every year) you just log in to your UpToDate® account and click on the CME hours accrued in the upper right hand corner and then follow the prompts. Credits are redeemed as AMA PRA Category 1 Credits. I never claim all that I accrue, but they are especially helpful if you're running behind on CME credits one year and realize last minute, or if you use it to boost your annual conference credits to get to your annual requirement. They are at no extra cost to you (it's included in your subscription).

There is a lot more detailed information regarding UpToDate® and its utility in the clinic, but I think the above is a great summary and I'm not looking to bore you to death with every detail. I'm just trying to highlight the best parts of it. A lot of my co-workers have used other apps and resources such as Epocrates® and Medscape and I'm not saying they're inadequate resources (I know my counterparts like them a lot), but I just don't have a lot of personal experience with them, so I won't go into detail about them. Just know they are out there to explore on your own.

OKPMP

This website in Oklahoma is: www.oklahoma.pmpaware.net. The "PMP" stands for prescription monitoring program. Most states have these now. Logging into this site is expected every time you write for a controlled substance (ie. opioids and benzodiazepines are the most common). It allows providers in Oklahoma to see what prescriptions have recently been written for a patient. You can see when the last time a controlled substance was prescribed, who it was written by (and their corresponding workplace address), the number of pills provided, and how long of a supply this was intended to be. Now, we can even search surrounding states' prescription monitoring programs to cut down on drug seeking and diversion behaviors. Each state is likely to have one of these monitoring programs and they are extremely beneficial.

"Your Birth Control Choices"

This is a handout that I routinely print and give to women who are considering their options for birth control. It is a very clear table, which describes the method, how it is used (implant in arm, inserted in uterus, inserted in vagina, pill taken by mouth, injection in arm, etc.), how well it works statistically, and the most common pros and cons. I find that a lot of women don't know that there are so many options available to them, and it is a great source to send home with them so they can review it after the visit. It is provided by www.reproductiveaccess.org.

False Positive Table

This one is crucial. As I mentioned before, an abnormal or unexpected urine drug screen result is never a pleasant finding. Instantly, I'm worrying about the patient blowing up on me when I ask about the inconsistency. Sometimes they fess up, but most of the time they are very offended and upset that I would question their integrity. This table was suggested to me by a pharmacist that I work with. I always call and confirm with pharmacy regarding unexpected UDS results to ensure there isn't a drug that they are taking that could be causing a false positive that I've missed. It is a great resource to look up the most common drugs that cause false positives. Again, when in doubt always send the sample for a confirmatory test. I usually, depending on my level of suspicion, will go ahead and renew whatever controlled medication I'm prescribing until I get a confirmed result, which demonstrates that the patient has deviated from our previous agreement. Then we have "the talk." The website is https://www.uspharmacist.com/article/urine-drug-screening-minimizing-false-positives-and-false-negatives-to-optimize-patient-care.

State Meth Registry

This is a useful tool that was also brought to my attention by a pharmacist I work with. At times I would order pseudoephedrine and per our in-house pharmacy policy we could not dispense pseudoephedrine to anyone who was registered in the state meth registry website. To access the site all you have to do is type in the patient's information (name and birthdate) and it tells you if they are a registered offender. Simple enough. The website https://obn-methcheck.appriss.com.

State immunization log (OSIIS)

Each state in which you practice will most likely have an online system that logs immunizations. In Oklahoma, where I practice, it is called Oklahoma State Immunization Information System (OSIIS). Here you can look up previous immunizations and log ones that patients have recently received. This is very helpful when patients get immunizations at various locations (health department, previous PCP office, other), but it only works when the immunizations are manually entered, and it is usually state-by-state. If someone received an immunization outside of Oklahoma, for example, it won't be in our system. For this reason, I still think it is a good idea for patients to keep their own paper record of immunizations, but it is somewhat helpful if consistently used. The website is https://osiis.health.ok.gov.

Catch-up vaccination scheduler

The vaccination scheduler is used to help determine a personalized vaccination timeline for a patient who is behind on vaccines. This is most helpful for pediatric patients who have gotten off schedule and usually it's used by nursing staff, but it's worth mentioning here. Here's how it works: First, you type in the patient's age and current vaccinations. Then, the system calculates when to give the next vaccine and the subsequent dates that the others can be given based on how long you must wait between injections. The website is https://www.vacscheduler.org.

App Resources

UpToDate®

We've already talked a lot about UpToDate® and you should download the app. End of story.

Shots

This is a fantastic app developed by the American Academy of Family Physicians and the Society of Teachers of Family Medicine. They used information from the CDC and the Advisory Committee on Immunization Practices to create this resource. The app is very helpful for quick access to immunization recommendations including schedules (for children and adults), catch-up schedules, and combination vaccines. It is organized by the appropriate schedule, or you can also search based on a specific condition the patient may have. Alternatively, you can search the specific vaccine and can then view recommendations, indications, and contraindications based on the vaccine in question. Lastly, you can actually create a patient profile with the patient's age, certain conditions/diagnoses, and social risk factors (such as military, health care worker, IV drug use, homelessness, etc.). Based on the characteristics you select, a list populates with the recommended vaccinations for that individual. It is a super valuable and easy to use resource with a lot of good information. I often tell nursing staff about it since they deal with a lot more of the day to day immunizations than I do.

Contraception

Get a contraception app. There are several out there and they generally have the same information. One trustworthy option would be the one created by the CDC. The information in this one is split up into two major sections: MEC (which stands for medical eligibility criteria) and SPR (selected practice recommendations for contraception use). The MEC section helps a provider determine whether it is considered safe to use a particular method of birth control. There is a nice chart of this on the CDC's website, but I didn't actually find it in the app. Instead, they ask you to select the patient's major medical problems and then it cross checks that information with the current recommendations and gives its rating: 1,2,3, or 4. One is "no restriction (method can be used)." Two is "advantages generally outweigh theoretical or proven risks." Three is "theoretical or proven risks usually outweigh the advantages." Four is "unacceptable health risk (method not to be used)." The SPR section helps providers troubleshoot problems or side effects that can be associated with various methods of birth control. It also gives information regarding when to start certain methods, how to switch between methods, proper follow up, etc. I generally use a contraception app every time I see someone to discuss a contraception method. There's a lot of information out there to know. Use your resources or you'll go insane.

MDCalc

This is an app that directs you to the www.mdcalc.com website. The website contains a ton of calculators including creatinine clearance, CHA2DS2-VASc, HAS-BLED, calcium correction for hypoalbuminemia, and on, and on. The information is separated into "Popular," "Favorites," "Specialty," "All," and "Guidelines." There is also a search bar to quickly find what you need. The resources I use most often are the calculators in the "Popular" section.

GoodRx

This app is essential for personal and patient use. I first learned about it when I was working in a free clinic, because we would use it to search for a particular drug our patient needed to see where he or she could get it the cheapest. You just type in the drug into the search box, and select the type of pill (capsule, tablet, etc.), and the quantity. Next, enter your zip code and it then displays the closest and cheapest options. The cheapest price includes their coupons, which you can easily save to "My Coupons" to show the pharmacy and get that lowest price.

There are also other great features on the app like refill reminders and price alerts, which notifies you if they find a cheaper price on a chronic medication. I've personally used this app to find the cheapest price for an antimalarial drug when I was preparing to move to Ecuador for a year. Because I was getting a whole year in advance I had to pay the cash price without any help from insurance. This app helped me find the cheapest place to get a 12-month supply. That savings really adds up!

Another fantastic feature is the pill identifier. This is so helpful in clinic when a patient says, "I think I had anaphylaxis with the blue blood pressure pill, but I don't remember what it's called…" Or consider using it when (not if) a patient brings his pills in a pill organizer, but no bottles with names, strengths, etc.

ePSS

This app is great for individualized recommendations for patients based on the USPSTF Preventive Services Database. Here's how it works: first you select the patient's age, sex, tobacco use, sexual activity, and whether the patient is pregnant or not. After entering your patient's information as above, it populates the current recommendations for your patient from the USPSTF. It organizes the results based on the rating of the recommendation (A, B, C, D, or I).

Additionally, you can search through all the resources on the site based on the counseling or screening you're interested in, such as breast cancer screening, or asymptomatic bacteriuria screening. You can also search based on whether it is a screening, counseling, or preventive measure you have a question about. Furthermore, you can bookmark certain guidelines you want to be able to quickly review later. They also have a ton of tools to print and use for screenings to give patients or guidelines to hang up in your office as reminders for you. This is definitely a must use tool.

ASCVD Plus

This is another must have in the clinic. It is used to calculate a patient's 10-year and lifetime risk of developing atherosclerotic cardiovascular disease. There are several guidelines that are based on this calculated risk percentage (for example statin and aspirin use). More than that, it is a useful tool to have discussions with patients, because based on the information you enter about the patient, you can choose to see what the risk reduction might be if you add a statin, add blood pressure medicine, stop smoking, etc. There is also a section for specific advice regarding each comorbidity, for example, blood pressure or aspirin guidelines. Lastly, there is a button to view all risk reduction scenarios which reveals what the risk would be given certain changes (add statin, stop smoking, etc.). In the advice section you can view a table, which lists out all of the information to consider with your patient during the shared-decision making discussion in checklist format.

ACS Risk Calculator

The official name of this app is: "ACS NSQIP Surgical Risk Calculator". I discovered this app at a conference during a talk about preoperative clearance. The physician giving the talk recommended this app to help determine risk of postoperative complications based on specific information. Here's how you use the app. First, you select the procedure the patient is considering having (for example elective laparoscopic cholecystectomy). Next, you enter other information regarding the patient (age, sex, functional status, steroid use, history of cancer, CHF, COPD, tobacco use, history of renal disease, etc.). Once the information is computed, there is a graphic that is colored green, yellow, or red (green for likely positive outcome or average risk for the given category, red for increased risk, and yellow for somewhere in between). There are several categories to consider including risk of serious complication, surgical site infection, pneumonia, venous thromboembolism, readmission, return to the OR, sepsis, and death, among others. On the graphic you can also compare the patient's calculated risk to the average risk in each category of potential complication. After the report is created you can email or print the report. It obviously is just an estimate of the risk given the patient's comorbidities, but it feels better than just sort of eyeballing a patient and their chart and then trying to determine his risk. I have found it to be useful in my practice.

Figure 1

This app is mostly for fun. It is essentially like a social media feed for medical providers. All the posts are about interesting clinical cases or questions. There are lots of pictures of astonishing bone fractures, brain MRIs, rashes, EKGs and lots more. It's a fun place to explore when you're looking for some interesting clinical cases to inspire you.

The Human Diagnosis Project

This one is also for fun, but even more than that it is for continued learning. Basically, it is a collection of clinical cases to work through and solve. First, you are given a few symptoms and then asked to provide a differential diagnosis. Next, you are given physical exam findings, pertinent imaging, and any other important information the patient may offer you. You are expected to update your differential after each new clue. At the end, the correct diagnosis is displayed along with what most other people diagnosed and a few important teaching points. I previously looked everywhere for a free resource to practice on virtual patient cases. Unfortunately, I didn't discover this app until a few years into practice while listening to "The Curbsiders" podcast, which I will discuss in more detail later.

This app significantly challenges my diagnostic skills in a very fun way. It's helpful to see what other people diagnosed and to see how they may have thought about things differently. Their purpose as stated on their app is to create an international effort to build an open intelligence system to help improve diagnostic accuracy and the overall health of patients. I love that the emphasis is on building your differential and ultimately reaching the correct diagnosis. A lot of resources focus on the correct treatment, but you can always look that up. Getting the correct diagnosis is sometimes much harder. Medicine is more gray than black and white. Nothing is textbook presentation, and this app can help sharpen your diagnostic skills.

Uncommon Sources of Continuing Medical Education Credits

Initially, I was worried about getting all the continuing medical education (CME) credits that my license and certification requires, but I've not found it to be an issue over the last several years. Currently, my certification through NCCPA requires me to acquire 100 credits over the span of two years with no other stipulations. However, my state license requires me to obtain 20 credits every year and at least one of those credits must be on the topic of substance abuse. My normal routine to satisfy these requirements is to obtain around 50 credits each year (one has to be in substance abuse each year). I normally attend a three day conference in person (worth 35 Category 1 CME credits), and then I supplement that with about 10-15 credits or so via my UpToDate® CME acquired on the job (previously discussed). The conference I attend annually is our Oklahoma Association of Physician Assistants, so they always make sure to build the one credit of substance abuse that is required into the lectures, so it is easy to fulfill this requirement if I attend that conference.

Additional CME can be earned via several methods: reading and answering questions from educational journals such as JAAPA, JNP, AAFP, etc., completing specialized training (medication assisted treatment, long acting reversible contraception, etc.), listening to certain podcasts that offer it, remote participation in a conference without your presence (purchase an audio recording and gain access to an online portal to answer questions), and my favorite method, which is purchasing the MKSAP series from the American College of Physicians (ACP). We'll discuss these in more depth next.

MKSAP

This is one of my absolute favorite methods of acquiring CME besides UpToDate®, because it's just so darn easy and you might as well be getting credit for all that work you're doing during your regular day in the clinic. MKSAP is a series of books and online resources that internal medicine residents often use to prep for their board exam. I was introduced to it on my internal medicine rotation in PA school. Every week the internal medicine residents (and so all of the medical and PA students) had a 2-3 hour evening meeting to discuss the previous week's MKSAP reading assignment and to review the clinical vignettes at the end of each chapter to test our knowledge. The MKSAP series comes in several options: print only, online only, or a combination of both. Because my employer pays for my MKSAP series I always opt for both, so that I have more options. Previously, I have almost exclusively utilized the online version to obtain CME credits. It works like this: first, you read through the chapter and when you come to the end of a section there are questions (clinical vignettes) regarding what you just read. Questions normally ask the "next best step" or "next best test," but there are also a lot of other types of questions to generally reinforce what you just read. After you finish reading and answering an entire subject (such as cardiology) you can claim your CME. I love that the questions in the online version come along while you read each short section instead of all at the end (like in the print version) for a few reasons. First, it is super helpful for me to apply and reinforce the information just after reading it. I believe this helps to increase retention. Also, in order to claim the CME credit for each section (which can be up to around 20 credits for a large section like cardiology) you have to correctly answer at least 50% of the questions. Because the question is just after the information, it increases your chances of getting the question right, so that you can claim your CME. Another important thing to know about the available CME is that there is a defined window of time allowed to claim it. Actually doing the claiming of it and downloading the certificate is easy, but it must be within the time window to do so. The last time I purchased it the CME was available for about a year. The MKSAP series allows you to get some serious CME on your own time and at your own pace without being required to travel for any conferences if you don't want to. It is an expensive program, so don't think you're going to be saving a lot up front using this resource instead of a physical conference. However, because of the large number of CME available, compared to a conference, it is somewhat cheaper in the end. Because of the intense interaction with the material and the ability to focus on a certain topic that you want to work on at that time, I think it is one of the best ways to obtain CME and really get a lot for your money.

There are also other ways of obtaining CME through the MKSAP series. If you get the "MKSAP Complete" (print and online) you also get some other resources such as "Board Basics," "Digital Flashcards," and "Virtual Dx." Board Basics is a great one-stop-shop for review on many topics. I believe it was intended to be a quick review of the more in-depth information found in each subject of the original expanded series. It is an all-in-one book (instead of the many volumes that make up the original). The Digital Flashcards program is also included in the "Complete" package. These are easily accessed (along with all the information contained in MKSAP) through an app on your phone. Flashcards on the go are always a good thing to have in your back pocket. The Virtual Dx is also another feature that is quite unique. It is an image-based self-assessment tool (with clinical vignettes) from which you can also obtain CME. This section was one of the last to expire when I used this before, so it is a good one to utilize and finish quickly (in order to claim your CME) if everything else is already expired. The ACP does email you to let you know that your CME will be expiring soon, and this is extremely helpful and appreciated.

Medication-Assisted Treatment

Another fantastic option for acquiring a significant amount of CME is to complete the "Medication-Assisted Treatment (MAT)" training online. Under the "Drug Addiction Treatment Act of 2000" NPs and PAs are legally allowed to write for buprenorphine for the indication of opioid dependence, after completing the required training. In order to receive the "waiver" to write for that indication, midlevels must complete 24 hours of online training modules. The first 8 hour training module is the same one required for physicians, and then an additional 16 hour training module is required for midlevels to receive their waiver. The training is provided by the Substance Abuse and Mental Health Services Administration which is associated with the U.S. Department of Health and Human Services. The modules (when I took the courses) were created by a combination of experts including midlevels and physicians. This training is COMPLETELY FREE and is worth a whopping 24 hours of CME credits (all are obviously on the topic of substance abuse, so if your licensing board requires any hours dedicated to that like mine does you're more than covered the year you complete this training). They also have a free app called MATx for treatment and prevention tools and resources for healthcare providers.

After you finish the training (consisting of several PowerPoints and questions at the end of each, which require a certain number of correct answers to pass), you have the option to apply for a "waiver." This waiver allows you to write for buprenorphine specifically for the indication of opioid dependence and you must have the training and waiver in order to legally write for this indication. Once you submit your application for the waiver, in about 45 days you will receive another DEA number. Don't worry, you don't have to pay another $750 for your new number; it is free. The new number (in my case) basically just changed the letters preceding my number to XR instead of MR. You actually use both letter-number combinations. You use the MR# for regularly scheduled drugs and the XR# when you write for buprenorphine for the indication of opioid dependence. I have found that being able to offer this service to patients has been very rewarding. Anytime you are working with patients and addiction you will probably experience a little more turbulence and difficulties at times, but I think the cause is totally worth it. I have had so many patients thank me multiple times during a visit for providing this service to them. They describe desperately wanting to get off of pain pills or heroin, but don't have the resources to go to a clinic far away or to one that they can't afford. A lot of patients know about buprenorphine and buprenorphine/naloxone medications and have actually taken them before (purchased off the street or from a friend). They can attest to the difference it makes in their life. Often they report that the buprenorphine/naloxone completely removed their craving for opioids. It also tends to help with pain without the high and brain fog that comes along with the other full agonist opioids like pain pills and heroin.

In addition to getting free CME, and helping a huge number of people regain their jobs, children, and lives (especially in our current time of opioid crisis), you can also use this free training to boost your resume and even get a hefty raise. When I completed my MAT training I received an annual increase in my salary of 5%, which ended up being around $5,000 per year. Not too bad for only 24 hours' worth of work (that's around $208 per hour). They make the process of requesting the waiver really easy, too. So, why not utilize this resource to further your education and specialization, help others immensely, and boost your income?! Are you sold yet? If so, here is the site to check out: https://pcssnow.org/medication-assisted-treatment.

LARC

Long-acting reversible contraception (LARC) has been more widely accepted by women recently. I know when I first considered getting an intrauterine device (IUD) in college, my mom truly frightened me about the potential (rare) harms that were a lot more common when she was a young woman. There was an IUD decades ago that was associated with increased pelvic infections, intrauterine implantation of the device, and uterine perforation. Since the early 1970s when this particular IUD was being aggressively marketed, we have had a lot of medial advancements and the new IUDs (both hormonal and nonhormonal) are considered safe and extremely effective for birth control. In addition to IUDs as a form of LARC, there are hormonal implants if the woman prefers it. These 4cm long rods are placed just under the skin on the medial aspect of the arm. Obviously, there are risks and benefits for all of these, but expanding on those isn't the purpose of this book.

When searching for LARC training I contacted a friend who recommended participating in a training at an OBGYN conference. She did this and had a great experience. This is certainly an option, although it is more expensive than the one she told me about next. In Oklahoma, there are state programs funded to help combat the rising trend of teen pregnancy. The organization I did my training through (Focus Forward Oklahoma) offered it completely free to clinicians who provide care to patients 18 years and younger in their practice. I work in family practice, so this worked for me. The organization partners with several local universities to provide the training space and the OBGYN specialists to give the training. All I had to do was email the organization that I was interested in attending the training and they sent me a confirmation of the time and place. The training was one whole day and consisted of about 4 hours of IUD training and 4 hours of Nexplanon® training. A

Merck representative must provide the Nexplanon® training and after you complete their training, you are registered in their system. This allows you to actually order the product. Both portions of this training were absolutely phenomenal. There was a lot of great information and resources (including templates and patient information handouts all of which were provided in a spiral-bound book to take back to the clinic). There was plenty of time for asking questions to the experts, and lots of hands on training, which obviously is essential to feeling confident when you go into your first procedure on a real person. We also were sent home with sample IUD training applicators (of several different brands, because of course they all have to be a little different-eyes rolling), a few practice 3D uteruses (nulliparous and parous), and a practice silicone arm and Nexplanon application device. After the training, I felt adequately prepared to go out and offer these services.

I didn't receive any CME hours for this, but I am betting that if you pay to do this training at a conference you will likely receive CME credits. Even though I didn't get any CME credits, this also was an opportunity to boost my salary. The training qualified for the 5% raise that I mentioned before for the MAT training. Unfortunately, I already received the 5% raise for the MAT waiver, so I couldn't receive both. It was poor timing on my part, but hooray for more experience and patient satisfaction. It is definitely nice to offer options to your patients. Sure, you can send them to GYN for these services, but sometimes the patient just prefers to have her own provider that knows her and that she trusts perform these procedures. Also, in my rural practice patients didn't want to drive over an hour to the big city for the GYN referral, and would prefer to have it done at their home clinic in the rural area where they live.

Podcasts

"The Curbsiders"

Okay, so I really only have one or two podcasts to recommend for CME and general enjoyment, but I'm sure there are a lot more out there. I was just so lucky to find these that I never looked anywhere else for more. You can get CME credits for both of these recommendations, although I have never personally done it. The CME is available through the American College of Physicians® (ACP). We'll discuss that in more detail shorty. First, let me recommend a thousand times over "The Curbsiders" internal medicine podcast. After finding this podcast I have never searched for another. The information is so up to date and digestible. It is very valuable and well worth the time to listen, especially if you have a commute or enjoy listening to audio while you're working out. The cast on this show is absolutely hilarious and pretty much every episode I find myself laughing out loud in my car on the way home. It is truly enjoyable and very engaging. It actually helps me to NOT fall asleep on my 1.25 hour drive home instead of putting me to sleep like some other podcasts or talk radio shows can do. Basically, it is made up of a cast of about three main people. These are physicians who work in varying practices, but mostly in the hospital and primary care setting. They interview various experts in different specialties about the best and most up to date and efficient way to diagnose, treat, and offer patient education information. The focus is usually on primary care topics that you see on a regular basis. Their claim to fame is that they are "The internal medicine podcast that uses expert interviews to bring you clinical pearls and practice changing knowledge." I find this statement to be profoundly true.

They have had many rotating guests in the past to help interview their experts. Their audience is made up of a wide variety of listeners:

Pre-Med students, medical students, PA and NP students, and practicing physicians and midlevels. Because they have such a broad listening base they ask the experts broad questions at first to help the audience get a feel for the background and general information first. This is helpful even for those who have been practicing for a while, because well you've been practicing for a while and have probably forgotten some of the basic foundational information you used to have memorized from your med school text. Then, they drill down on the relevant specifics and focus the episodes to discuss actionable recommendations and guidelines. The episodes are usually about 30-60 minutes long which is perfect for my long drive home. I hate wasting that 2.5 hours of my day, so listening to these informational podcasts helps me to not waste time and also stay up to date on the most current medical information. I have on repeated occasions listened to an episode and then a couple days later had a patient with a complaint or question related to what I had listened to. I was able to take information discussed in the episode and use it to bolster my conversation with my patient. Did I mention you can get CME for listening to this radio gold? See the next section for details on how.

"Core IM"

This podcast is also great and deserves a mention. It is also an internal medicine podcast supported by the American College of Physicians (ACP) and can be utilized to acquire CME credits. It is produced by several physicians who focus on keeping the information clear and concise. They also try to design these episodes to facilitate repetition and retention of knowledge, so that you are able to recall the information when you have a patient in front of you. When I first listened to it the episodes were fairly short (15-20 minutes), which helped me to keep my focus throughout the whole episode. Now, I have recently found several longer episodes (around 45 minutes). They focus on reinforcing information via quizzes at the beginning and end. They also use relatively new techniques to help reinforce information from previous episodes such as spaced repetition, which has been shown to help improve retention. They have been featured on "The Curbsiders" podcast described above. After you listen to an episode of "The Curbsiders" or "Core IM" you can take a quiz on ACP's website and then claim the CME. One hour of audio is worth about one credit. There are also transcripts of the episodes and general information about each podcast on ACP's website. Another podcast that you can listen to and get CME is "Annals On Call." This is a podcast hosted by Dr. Bob Centor and a rotating expert who together discuss an interesting and often controversial article that has recently been published in the Annals of Internal Medicine. These CME credits are free to members of ACP.

Salary, Benefits, and Other Information

When I interviewed for my first job I had no idea what salary I should expect and what benefits were generally offered. I remember scrambling trying to talk to all my friends from PA school to compare offers to figure out if mine was a good one or if I should keep looking. My hope is that sharing some of my own information with you will help give you an idea what is customary to offer. Of course every location, specialty, and setting will be different and therefore bring different offers, so remember that while reading. At least you will have some idea, because I had no clue.

First, I worked as a hospitalist PA at a rural hospital (not a level one trauma center). My starting salary was $99,885 as a new graduate with no experience and they offered a 2% raise annually up to a max of a $110,000 annual salary. We also had incentives, which could be earned by certain productivity measures, that equaled $2,500 per quarter (so $10,000 per year if each was earned). CME dollars that could be spent equaled $2,500 per year and they also covered the cost of my: state license, fee to maintain my NCCPA certification, DEA license, and OBNDD license. I didn't really have paid time off as a hospitalist, because we worked 7 days on and 7 days off (10 hour days). They considered our 7 days off our vacation time, so if we needed other days off or were sick we had to work it out with other coworkers to cover for us. Then, we had to either make that time up for a regular paycheck or just take a pay cut that pay period.

Lastly, they paid for my malpractice insurance. While we're on the subject of malpractice insurance let me say this: don't forget to read the fine print. There are two main types of medical malpractice insurance: occurrence and claims-made. The claims-made insurance only covers a suit that is filed WHILE you currently have that specific insurance. So, essentially when you leave that job and get different malpractice insurance you no longer have coverage over any of the patient encounters that you had with your previous employer. If someone files a claim on you within the statute of limitations, but after you have dropped that insurance (for example when you leave the job that is paying for it on your behalf), you have no coverage or representation. In contrast, occurrence insurance will cover any suit that may be brought up against you even after you leave your job and drop their coverage. In order to have coverage after you leave a job that has claims-made insurance you must pay for tail insurance. Long story short: occurrence coverage is better and you should try to get your employer to pay for this type.

My second job was in primary care working with a tribal Indian health facility. I'll first say that tribal facilities tend to pay better than federal IHS facilities, so keep that in mind when considering a position and what I will say next. My starting salary was $115,000. As described previously, I was able to increase this by obtaining further certifications including MAT and LARC training. This increased my salary by 5% (which ended up being a little more than $5,000 per year). Also, I was told that I should receive a 2-5% increase annually in my base pay depending on my annual review. They offered $5,000 per year in CME allowance in addition to purchasing my licenses as above, and also a new stethoscope (worth approximately $150). This amount of CME was what the physicians were offered at my hospital job. In addition to the great salary (especially for primary care) they also offered loan repayment. I did not have to apply for it through the government (which is an option if you work for a federal or tribal Indian health facility). This meant it was guaranteed as part of my benefits package. This is HUGE. When you apply for this benefit through the government you may or may not be granted the loan repayment. It depends on the number of applicants that year and also the need of the community that you're serving. They have a system to identify each town with a number, which indicates it's particular state of need. Not only was my loan repayment guaranteed, but I also didn't have to sign an agreement to serve for a certain amount of time. This is ever bigger. Usually it is a two-year commitment and if you don't complete the two years of service you must RETURN your loan repayment! I never liked the idea of being trapped in a certain position, especially when you don't even know what the work environment will be like.

Regarding time off, my primary care job included 260 hours of PTO. I worked 10-hour days at that time, so this was a whopping 26 days days off per year (totaling 6.5 weeks PTO since we worked 4 days per week). That was in addition to national and tribal holidays, which totaled approximately 15 more days off. When I was deciding whether to switch jobs from the hospital to the clinic, this definitely factored in. After doing the math, this primary care job (which was 4 days per week working 10 hour days) was actually less total days at work than my hospital job working 7 days on and 7 days off.

In addition to the generous PTO and holidays, we also had a significant amount of administrative time to complete notes and notifications. This is not the norm. Most clinic hours are 8 AM to 5 PM, five days per week, and you get your work done during that time or on your own time. I was very fortunate to have an entire morning (5 hours) every week to get caught up on notes and notifications (reviewing labs, notes from specialists, placing orders, etc.). This really allowed me to get my work done at work and not take any home. Although, it was sort of a trade off because of the long drive to get to work. Part of the reason the benefits were so great at this tribal clinic was because they had to make their package attractive and extraordinary, because it was about an hour and a half away from the city.

Lastly, make sure you are a member of your national organization (AANP and AAPA). AAPA has an annual report and the AANP does also. AAPA releases a salary report every year with all kinds of information regarding the percent of PAs who work in each specialty, the average salary, average number of hours worked per week, general satisfaction in each specialty, along with a lot of other useful information. If you are being underpaid or overworked you can take this information to your employer and try to negotiate changes to your contract or working schedule. You must be a member to get these reports for free, but if you don't want to be a member for some reason you can purchase them. This is the best information I can give you based on my own personal experience. These are only two examples and they will become outdated quickly, so expect to hear about a lot of other benefit packages that may be dissimilar. I still encourage you to talk with your friends and coworkers to determine what the most competitive package is for you based on your own values.

Most common ___________

In this section, I originally planned on providing the most common reasons for office visits, and their appropriate algorithm, table, etc. However, this information will always be changing and you'll develop your own favorite tables and algorithms. So, instead, my goal for this section is to give you a list of the most common problems, lab abnormalities, and patient education handouts that I normally give, so that you can have a little bit of a head start. My recommendation would be to take these "most common" lists, and then use your favorite resource from our previous discussion to further plan your next steps. Use resources you love and create bookmarks, printouts, hyper-links on your desktop, or whatever other means that is most convenient to you so that you can have this information readily available to address when the time comes.

Most common problems:

1. Plantar fasciitis
2. Musculoskeletal pain in general (back, knee, shoulder, ankle)
3. Abdominal pain
4. Diabetes
5. Hypertension
6. Contraception
7. Epidermoid Cyst
8. Viral syndrome
9. Insomnia
10. Urinary tract infection
11. Fatigue
12. Orthostatic hypotension
13. Pain management
14. Acute otitis externa
15. Acute otitis media
16. Non-alcoholic fatty liver disease
17. Contact dermatitis
18. Eczema
19. Allergic rhinitis
20. Opioid dependence
21. Coronary artery disease
22. Hyperlipidemia
23. Cellulitis
24. Paronychia
25. General physical (sports, work, other)
26. Seborrheic and actinic keratoses, nevus, solar lentigo, skin tag
27. Dizziness
28. Anxiety
29. Depression
30. Lower extremity swelling
31. Herpes simplex virus or other sexually transmitted infection
32. Low testosterone
33. Migraines
34. Breast lump
35. Simple laceration

Most common lab abnormalities:

1. Hypokalemia
2. Elevated transaminases
3. Elevated alkaline phosphatase
4. Elevated white blood cell count
5. Elevated or reduced hemoglobin
6. High or low mean corpuscular volume (MCV)
7. Elevated A1c
8. Elevated or low thyroid stimulating hormone (TSH, T4)
9. Reduced kidney function
10. Sodium abnormality
11. Low testosterone
12. Low iron
13. Elevated blood urea nitrogen (BUN)
14. Elevated or low patelets
15. Low vitamin D
16. Elevated lipids
17. Elevated microalbumin
18. Bacteriuria

Most common patient education:

1. Hepatitis C
2. Tendinitis (bicep and rotator cuff)
3. Plantar fasciitis
4. Ingrown Toenail
5. Contraception information

List of Materials Needed for Common Procedures

The following lists are intended to help you more quickly gather materials for common procedures in the primary care setting. I have a folder on my desk full of sticky notes that I search through when needed to quickly find the materials we need for any given procedure. I felt it would be helpful to offer you the lists here, so you can print them and have them handy for your practice. During minor procedures I always play the patient's favorite genre of music to help lighten the mood. They always laugh when I ask what their favorite music is and they generally seem to enjoy the procedure better.

Ingrown toenail removal:

· 10mL 1% lidocaine plain (with 18g needle to draw this up)

· 25g need for performing digital block

· Alcohol swabs

· Iodine swabs

· Ethyl chloride spray

· Nail lifter

· Nail clipper

· Hemostat

· Gauze

· Silver nitrate or phenol

Insertion of Nexplanon®:

· Ruler or tape measure
· Surgical marker
· Iodine swabs
· Sterile gloves
· 2mL of 1% lidocaine plain in 3mL syringe with 1.5" 25g needle
· Nexplanon applicator device
· Sterile gauze
· Sterile bandage
· Pressure dressing materials (gauze and self-adherent wrap like Coban™)

Removal of Nexplanon®:

- Surgical marker
- Iodine swabs
- 1mL of 1% lidocaine plain in 3mL syringe and 1" 25g needle
- Sterile gauze
- Sterile bandage
- Pressure dressing materials (gauze and self-adherent wrap like Coban™)

Simple suture:

· Appropriate suture for location and depth

· Hemostat

· Scissors

· Sterile gloves

· Sterile saline to wash site

· 1% lidocaine with or without epi depending on site

Joint injection:

· Look up: "Intraarticular and soft tissue injections: What agent(s) to inject and how frequently?" from UpToDate®

· Appropriate amounts of steroid and anesthetic as above (triamcinolone and lidocaine are common)

IUD insertion:

- Water-based lubricant
- Speculum
- Iodine swabs
- Tenaculum
- Uterine sound
- IUD
- Curved blunt scissors

IUD removal:

- Water-based lubricant
- Speculum
- Sponge forceps

Templates

Below are a few of the templates I created for myself to help write my notes more quickly and also to help me remember several important aspects of these visits. These are certainly customizable, and are intended only to be a guide. I may have left out certain elements of these visits, so please use your own judgment when interviewing, examining, and treating patients.

MASTER SHEET TEMPLATE

Problems today:
1) 2)

Problems for next time:
1) 2)

HPI:
Chronic problems:

Today's problem:

Objective

Vital signs:

Preventive care:

• Last PAP: ________	Result: ________	Next due: ________
• Last mammogram: ________	Result: ________	Next due: ________
• Last colonoscopy / other: ________	Result: ________	Next due: ________
• Last PSA if desired: ________	Result: ________	Next due: ________
• Last DEXA: ________	Result: ________	Next due: ________

Immunizations:	UTD:
• Flu q 1 year	________
• Td booster q 10 years	________
• Pneumococcal ≥65 years old (PCV13 then PPSV23 one year later)	________
• Zoster vaccine ≥60 years old	________

Physical Exam:
Pertinent findings:

Assessment/Plan:

1.
2.
3.
4.
5.

Diagnosis:

Treatment plan:

Medication changes:

Other instructions:

Next visit:

MASTER SHEET TEMPLATE EXAMPLE

Problems today:
1) *Heartburn* 2)

Problems for next time:
1) 2)

HPI:
Chronic problems:

65 year old male with a PMHx of COPD, CAD s/p CABG x 3, DM2, GERD, BPH, OA

Today's problem:

Heartburn worse over last month
Pain in LUQ x 30-60 minutes after dinner every night
Taking TUMS in addition to his ranitidine
Eats a lot of spicy foods and is on daily meloxicam for OA
3/10 on pain scale when present
No history of GI bleed or PUD

Objective

Vital signs:

Preventive care:

• Last PAP: ________	Result: ________	Next due: ________
• Last mammogram: ________	Result: ________	Next due: ________
• Last colonoscopy *2015*	Result: *normal*	Next due: *2025*
• Last PSA if desired: *deferred*	Result: ________	Next due: ________
• Last DEXA: ________	Result: ________	Next due: ________

Immunizations:	UTD:
• Flu q 1 year	✓
• Td booster q 10 years	✓
• Pneumococcal ≥65 years old (PCV13 then PPSV23 one year later)	✓
• Zoster vaccine ≥60 years old	✓

Physical Exam:
Pertinent findings:

LUQ pain

Assessment/Plan:
1. *GERD; + omeprazole 20mg daily*
2.
3.
4.

Diagnosis:

GERD: uncontrolled reflux/heartburn

Treatment plan:

Start omeprazole 20mg at night
Don't eat 30-60 minutes before to bed
Avoid spicy foods, carbonated and caffeinated drinks, acidic foods (like tomatoes)
Take TUMS or other antacid as needed

Medication changes:

Start omeprazole 20mg at night

Other instructions:

Next visit:

Follow up in one month if things aren't better.
If heartburn gets better then return for general follow up in 6 months.

GENERAL EXAM TEMPLATE

Subjective

HPI:

Chronic problems:

Today's problem:

Objective

Vital signs from visit here

Preventive care:

•Last PAP:	Result:	Next due:
•Last mammogram:	Result:	Next due
•Last colonoscopy/other:	Result:	Next due:
•Last PSA if desired:	Result:	Next due:
•Last DEXA:	Result:	Next due:

Immunizations:

•Flu q 1 year	Date given:	Next due:
•Td booster q 10 years	Date given:	Next due:
•Pneumococcal >65 years old (PCV13 then PPSV23 one year later)	Date given:	Next due:
•Zoster vaccine >60 years old	Date given:	

Physical Exam:

General: pleasant; in no apparent distress

HEENT: normocephalic, atraumatic; extraocular muscles intact; canals clear bilaterally; tympanic membrane translucent without erythema bilaterally; pharynx without erythema or exudate; no tonsillar enlargement; no cervical lymphadenopathy; without thyroid enlargement or nodule

Skin: clean and dry, without significant rash or wound

Cardiovascular: regular rate and rhythm; without appreciable murmur; without lower extremity bilaterally

Respiratory: clear to auscultation bilaterally; without wheeze, rhonchi, or rales

Abdominal: bowel sounds present, soft, nontender to palpation

Musculoskeletal: moves all extremities; gait normal

Assessment/Plan:

Well Woman Exam Template:

HPI:

Gyn Hx:
history of D&C or C-section

family history of breast, uterine, or ovarian cancer

Menstrual Hx:
- menarche: age
- LMP:
- cycle length:
- menstrual regularity:
- bleeding days:
- # pads/tampons:
- clots:
- intermenstrual bleeding:

Contraception use:
- previous:
- current:

Screening Hx:
- history of sexual infections
- number of lifetime partners (or # in last 2 months):
- discharge, itching, sores, pain with sex, bleeding after sex
- last pap: result:
- last mammogram: result:
- last colonoscopy: result:

OB Hx:
- G_P_ _ _ _
- year
- type of delivery
- complications
- spontaneous vs. induced abortions

Well Woman Exam Template Continued:

Physical Exam:
Vital signs from visit here

Gen: pleasant in NAD
HEENT: normocephalic, atraumatic; EOMI; canal clear; TM translucent without erythema b/l; pharynx without erythema or exudate; no tonsillar enlargement; no cervical lymphadenopathy; without thyroid enlargement or nodule
Skin: clean and dry, without significant rash or wound
CV: RRR; without appreciable murmur; without lower extremity edema b/l
Resp: CTAB; without wheeze, rhonchi, or rales
Abd: bowel sounds present, soft, NTTP

Breasts: symmetrical, without any skin changes, tenderness, masses, dimpling, or discharge

Pelvic Exam:
Vulva: w/o lesions, w/o bartholin or skene gland enlargement; urethra WNL
Vagina: pink and rugated; physiologic discharge present; no lesions; w/o cystocele
Cervix: no lesions; w/o cervical motion tenderness

Bimanual:
Uterus: firm, mobile, anteverted; NTTP
Adnexa: did not appreciate any adnexal masses or tenderness; ovaries palpable; normal size

Assessment/Plan:

Well Child Exam Template:

HPI:
No recent ER/Urgent Care visits since last appointment.
Home environment:
Education/Employment:
Eating habits:
Activities:
Drug use:
Sexuality:
Suicide/Depression:
Safety:

ROS:
Gen: no weight loss, weakness, fever, fatigue, or allergies
Skin: no rashes, itchiness, or bruising
HEENT: no vision problems, trouble hearing, hx of ear infections, discharge, pulling at ears, rhinorrhea, congestion, dysphagia, or speech problems
CV: no hx murmurs, anemia, turning blue, swelling in arms or legs
Resp: no trouble breathing, coughing, or wheezing
GI: normal bowel movements, no N/V/D
GU:
  F: menses onset, amt. duration, freq., pain, discharge, breast development
  M: puberty onset, erections, pain, discharge, swelling or pain in testes
MSK: no weakness, balance issues, muscle pain, swelling, or red/painful joints
Neuro: no brain or head injuries, seizures, fainting, dizziness, or numbness
Psych: no learning problems, difficulty with attention span, or hyperactivity

Objective

Vital signs from visit here

Physical Exam:

Gen: pleasant in NAD

HEENT: normocephalic, atraumatic; EOMI; canal clear; TM translucent without erythema b/l; pharynx without erythema or exudate; no tonsillar enlargement; no cervical lymphadenopathy

Skin: clean and dry, without significant rash or wound

CV: RRR; without appreciable murmur; 2+ femoral pulses b/l

Resp: CTAB; without wheeze, rhonchi, or rales

Abd: bowel sounds present, soft, NTTP

MSK: MAE; gait normal; spine straight; scapulae and iliac crests equal

GU: tanner stage

Neuro: 2+ brachioradialis, patellar, and achilles reflexes b/l

Assessment/Plan:

Anticipatory guidance given

All Resources:

Books:

1. The Sanford Guide to Antimicrobial Therapy 2019 by David Gilbert, M.D., et al.
2. Injection Techniques in Musculoskeletal Medicine A Practical Manual for Clinicians in Primary and Secondary Care by Stephanie Saunders and Steve Longworth
3. Clinician's Guide to Laboratory Medicine by Samir P. Desai, M.D.
4. Instant Work-Ups by Theodore X. O'Connell
5. Pocket Primary Care 2nd Edition by Meghan M. Kiefer and Curtis R. Chong

Websites:

1. UpToDate®: https://www.uptodate.com/home
2. OKPMP: www.oklahoma.pmpaware.net
3. Contraception choices: https://www.reproductiveaccess.org/wp-content/uploads/2014/06/contra_choices.pdf
4. False positive table: https://www.uspharmacist.com/article/urine-drug-screening-minimizing-false-positives-and-false-negatives-to-optimize-patient-care
5. Meth registry: https://obn-methcheck.appriss.com/
6. OSIIS: https://osiis.health.ok.gov
7. Catch-up vaccination scheduler: https://www.vacscheduler.org

Apps:

1. UpToDate®
2. Shots
3. Contraception
4. MDCalc
5. GoodRx
6. ePSS
7. ASCVD Plus
8. ACS Risk Calculator
9. Figure 1
10. The Human Diagnosis Project

CME:

1. MKSAP (by ACP)
2. Medication-Assisted Treatment: https://pcssnow.org/medication-assisted-treatment/
3. Long-acting reversible contraception

Podcasts:

1. The Curbsiders
2. Core IM
3. Annals On Call

Acknowledgements

I would like to give a special thanks to my loving husband, Dusty, who fully supported me when I told him about my wild dream to write a book. This book wouldn't exist without him. Thank you.

Made in United States
North Haven, CT
04 November 2026

21764040R00046